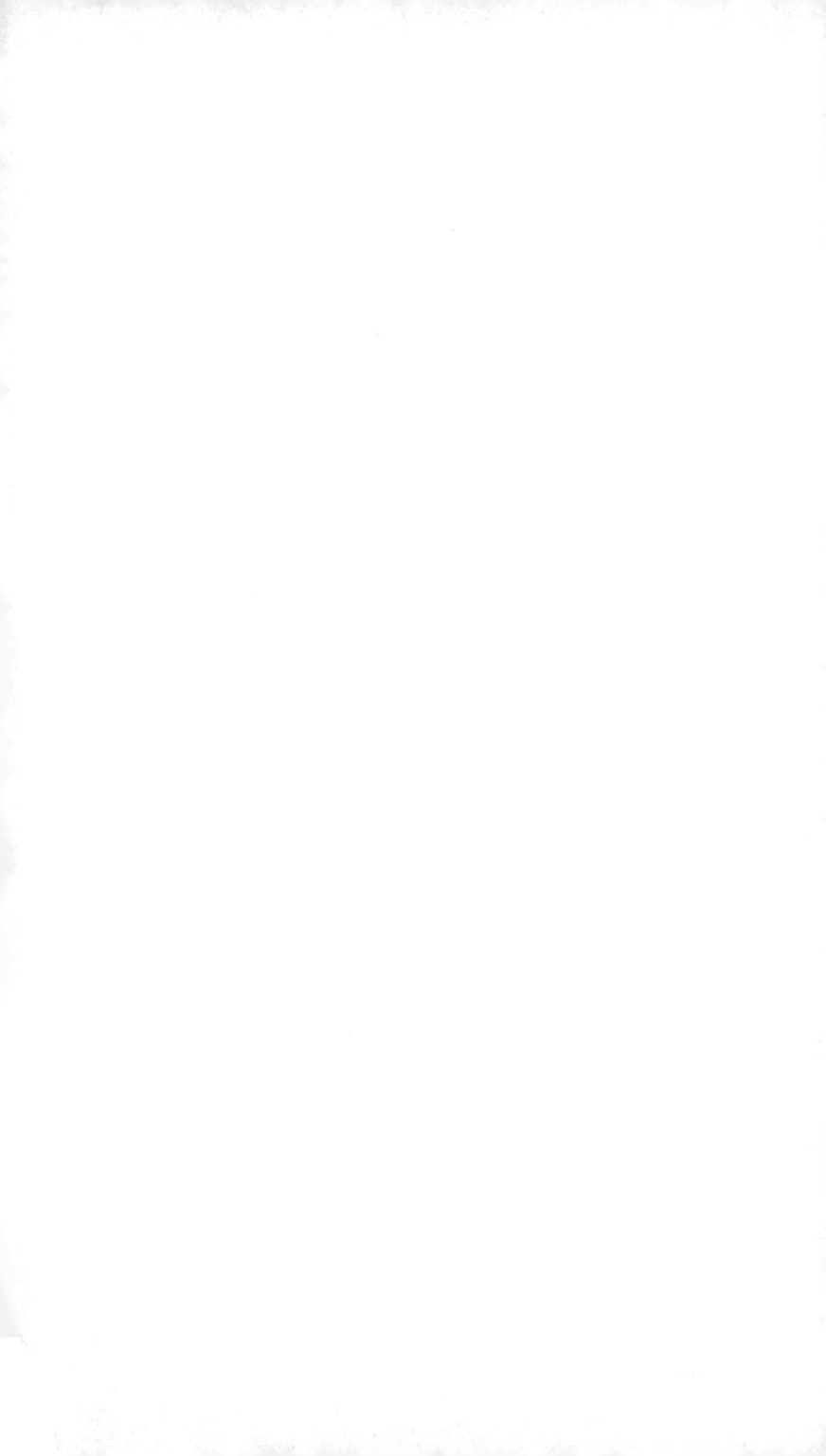

Cancer A Love Story

Thomas Lucas
and Suzanne Gallen-Lucas in spirit

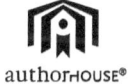
authorHOUSE®

AuthorHouse™
1663 Liberty Drive
Bloomington, IN 47403
www.authorhouse.com
Phone: 1-800-839-8640

First published by AuthorHouse 10/30/2009

ISBN: 978-1-4490-2704-9 (e)
ISBN: 978-1-4490-1248-9 (sc)

Printed in the United States of America
Bloomington, Indiana

This book is printed on acid-free paper.

I decided to write this story after three years of hell on earth to let couples know that if your loved one is diagnosed with a fatal form of cancer like Suzanne was, the only way you can help your spouse is to love him or her even more!

This story was completed on July 12, 2009, a year and a half after my wife, Suzanne, passed away from a rare form of ovarian cancer. Before that time I could not bring myself to tell our story to the rest of the world. In an effort to help others in the same situation or possibly console others, I decided to write this story. I hope it helps others manage the worst disease one can be afflicted with. This book is a mix of a love story, a biography, and a guide for how to support your loved one if he or she has cancer. This book may not be copied or sold except with permission of the author, Thomas Lucas.

Dedication

This book is dedicated to my loving wife, best friend, and soul mate. To her daughters, brothers, and sister. To my sons, my mother, my best friend, and the nurses and doctors who made her life less painful. To all couples who have had to traverse the great divide of a spouse who died from cancer.

Preface

This story is written from the time Suzanne developed cancer until she died on November 13, 2007. I know she is in a better place, and she still guides my life to this day. I never go to sleep without saying, "Good night, my love," and I look up to the stars and blow her a kiss.

Several years ago I bought Sue a teddy bear half the size of the other bear I also bought. I told Sue that the smaller bear was her and the big bear was me and I called them Squish and Squishy because of the way I hugged her. The teddy bears remain on my bed to this day, and when I feel alone, I pick up the small teddy bear and hug her and kiss her and tell her how much I miss her and love her, and sometimes I hear her say, "I will always love you, Tommy." That assumes you believe in spirits.

This story is true to form just the way it happened. Some sections of this story are heartbreaking, so be ready to cry, but you must also understand that Sue was the love of my life and that when we knew she was not going to make it I took a leave of absence from work to be her caregiver 24/7 for three months during the worst period of her life and mine as well. One day while Sue was lying on the couch in the living room she sat up and said to me, "Tommy, I can't take it anymore. I want to die." To hear someone as strong as Suzanne say those words to me was devastating. I hugged her and cried, and she just said one more phrase. "I love you, Tommy, and I could not have made it this far without you by my side. Thank you for loving me."

Suzanne died in the hospice ward of Abington Hospital with me and her children by her side. Suzanne did not want any fanfare, so she was cremated. I remember standing by the crematory with my best friend, Anthony, my brother, and his wife. Sue was in a cardboard box, and as the gentleman from the funeral parlor rolled the box to the crematory, I asked him to stop and open the box.

He said to me, "You know she has not been embalmed."

I said, "I want to see her one last time."

He said, "Be prepared. She does not look like you remember."

I said, "Open the box."

He did and said, "I will leave you alone for a few minutes."

There was no Suzie as I remember her in the box, just skin and bones. She weighed about seventy-five pounds. Her beautiful face was sunken in at the cheeks, her eyes were closed, and she smelled as though she was rapidly decaying. My brother said a prayer. I said nothing. I knew her soul was already with God, so I just looked at her with tears in my eyes and gave her a kiss and said, "I still love you, baby, and I will always love you for all eternity." When I received her remains I cried again, and to this day they are in an urn on a table in my apartment surrounded by two angels, and I sometimes place flowers next to her. She loved getting flowers, and sometimes I would hear her say, "They are beautiful," and I would say, "Yes, my love, just like you."

Contents

Chapter 1
Sue and Tom Are Happily Married

Sue and I were a typical middle-class couple. I had been working in the pharmaceutical industry for twenty-plus years. I was at the senior director level, and Sue was working for a small pharmaceutical company as the group manager. I say typical because we did everything other couples did—visited friends, went to the movies, went food shopping, cleaned house, took care of the bills, went to family parties, and took trips to Connecticut to see my mother. Sue's mom and dad passed away years ago. I was divorced from my first wife and then met Sue, the love of my life. We clicked immediately. She had three daughters and I had two sons, so at holidays our house was full. We had been married for nine years at this point in our relationship.

This period in time was when the pharmaceutical industry was losing money because of a lack of new drugs. There were new mergers going on every month, and people were losing their jobs so that the pharmaceutical industry could lower their head count and save money. Then came the acquisitions, and so I had to jump from one company to another, so we moved around from one county to another. However, because of my sons and Sue's daughter, who were all working, we tried to stay near our family. My wife was a very smart women, and she read book after book. She even asked me to explain what I did for a living, and I had to teach her about physiology. It really was not that bad because when I came home from work she wanted to know how my day went and Sue would come up with suggestions if I had a problem at work.

Regardless of various problems couples have to face from time to time, Sue and I were a team and managed problems together. Sue was my best friend, my lifelong companion, and a wonderful wife; we helped each other when we were down. Sue had a great personality was liked by almost everybody who met her. She was a strong individual who managed to overcome her very screwed-up childhood. We were happy and doing fine until she scheduled her yearly gynecology exam.

Chapter 2
Just a Routine Gynecologic Exam

In March of 2005 my wife went to have a routine gynecologic exam and physical and of course a Pap smear. Instead of going to her old physician, whom she trusted and had been seeing most all her life, Sue decided to go to a lab that was close to our home. My comment was that a Pap smear was a Pap smear and you couldn't screw that up. Boy was I wrong. After two weeks we found out that the Pap smear was abnormal. I immediately called the lab and told them who I was. I told them I was Dr. Thomas Lucas and my wife was Suzanne Gallen-Lucas and asked them to give me the results of the Pap smear. The lab tech told me that some of the cells on the smear were distorted and did not look typical.

I said, "How often do you find this kind of result, and what does it mean?" The tech's comment was "Not often," and the tech did not have experience with that type of cell before.

I said to Sue, "You should have gone to your old doctor."

The lab said they would repeat the study and get back to me in about two weeks. I was not happy about their time frame. When cancer is diagnosed, it is critical to move as fast as possible to get all the medical data and start chemo if it is appropriate. Some forms of cancer can spread very quickly depending on the type of cancer it is. Sue managed the possibilities in her head while I was anxious and could not think about anything but the thought that it could be *cancer*; I always think of the worst scenario first. That is just me. I called the lab back and asked them why it would take two more weeks to get the results, and the lab said it would take two more weeks to get the pathology report because the cells were atypical for cancer and they had not seen this abnormal type of cell before and needed to get a second opinion.

Those two weeks were agony for me, and I tried to hide my fear from Sue, but Sue knew me too well and knew I was dying inside waiting for the results. I would call the pathology lab three times a week and say, "This is Dr. Tom Lucas. Do you have the final report on my wife, Suzanne Gallen-Lucas?"

The answer was, "We cannot determine what kind of cells we are looking at, and we sent a sample to the University of Penn Medical College."

I was a little angry with their results and said, "It took you a month to decide you did not know what you were looking at and had to send it off to another Path lab? Remind me to forget to pay your bill until a month after I get it," and I hung up the phone.

I immediately called an associate of mine at Penn and asked him when we would get the results. He said, "Tom, I should have the info for you in about a week."

That was the longest week of my life while my wife just stayed cool, calm, and collected. She did not have my medical background, and I have to admit when something may medically be wrong with my wife I want the answer ASAP. When it comes the possibility of finding cancer in a loved one, time is of the essence. The sooner it is treated, the greater the chance you could have to go into remission. I hope whoever is reading this book realizes that there are very few types of cancer that can be cured even in this day and age. As an aside, based on my medical background, never get a gynecologic exam any place other than a university hospital, such as the University of Penn or Thomas Jefferson Medical center, to name a few. This is just my opinion.

This was just the beginning of three years of hell on earth, and here I was falling apart at the thought of losing the love of my life, my soul mate, to cancer. I had a feeling our life was going to change forever, but I kept those feelings to myself. I had to be strong for her and forced myself to be as positive as possible.

I said to Sue one day that if it was cancer, we would beat it. I told her I would get in touch with the most renowned oncologist in the United States and we would get a second opinion. Then I said, "I can take you to the top cancer centers in the United States. Do not worry, you will have the best oncologists, the latest treatments, and we will beat this ravaging disease."

I called the Mayo Clinic, MD Anderson, and Mass General. I knew some key opinion leaders in the field of cancer at these hospitals, and every one of them said, "Tom, I would be glad to have my team review your wife's chart."

This may sound arrogant on my part calling all of these experts I worked with in the past. I know, but this was my wife we were talking about, and I was a senior director with a pharmaceutical company with thirty years of clinical drug development experience under my belt. I had a master's degree in pharmacology and a PhD in medical physiology. Although I was not an MD, I spent thirty years studying medicine and had taken a sixty-hour course in cancer at Harvard University in 1989.

I realized that I was a little behind the times, but you can bet that almost once a week I spent hours reading and analyzing the latest information , research studies, and drugs for the treatment of ovarian cancer, which I thought it was. I started to make Suzie crazy. I asked her if she wanted to go to Texas to the MD Anderson Cancer center or the Dana Farber Institute in Massachusetts or Fox Chase or Thomas Jefferson University Hospital.

I was losing it. I forced myself to calm down, and while we were waiting for the second pathology report I came up with a plan.

As an aside to couples having to deal with a loved one who has been diagnosed with cancer, my advice would be to take it one step at a time. Do not fear what is still unknown, and for God's sake, do not make it worse on your spouse like I did without having the results. Schedule a consult with your gynecologist before you decide what to do next. Well, finally I received a call from the University of Penn.

"Dr. Lucas, Tom, we saw something on the Pap test, and we are sure it is a rare form of cancer called primary peritoneal cancer, a form of ovarian cancer."

I was devastated when I heard the news. I had one of the hardest tasks of my life. I had to tell my wife that she had cancer. Sue came home from work that day, and she could see the tears in my eyes and said to me, "You got the results."

I said, "Yes, my love, I have."

I sat her down on the couch hugged her and cried. I must have kissed her at least ten times, and Sue, being as strong of a person as she was, said, "Tommy." She called me Tommy from time to time. Until I met her only my mother called me Tommy. "Try and calm down and tell me what the results were from the Pap smear," she said.

I said, "Sue, you have ovarian cancer."

She was silent. She looked at me and said, "Now what?" That just goes to show you how strong of a women Sue was.

I said, "We need to decide on a cancer center and send them the Pap smear data and make an appointment to speak with their best cancer oncologist."

Sue said to me, "Well, I trust you, and wherever you want to take me is fine with me." Sue then said, "Now calm down. Remember what you said to me before. We will beat this."

I said, "Sue, I am sorry I am acting like a scared rabbit, but you know how much I love you, and I cannot accept the possibility that you could die."

Sue just looked at me and said, "Remember what we said. We can beat this." Sue repeated the phrase, and her strength made me feel a little better.

I said, "You're right, we can beat this."

Two days later I told Sue I wanted her to see a doctor at a cancer center that has a good reputation and was outside of Philadelphia. I told her that I made some phone calls to past associates and they said that this cancer center had a doctor who was very good and that he was a surgical oncology gynecologist.

Sue said, "Tommy, what is his name?"

I said, "His name is Dr. Larry Harper. I checked his credentials, and he is an MD and is board certified in oncology and gynecology as well as being a board-certified surgeon." For those who might be reading this story, the above is not the doctor's real name, for obvious reasons.

A week later we went to see Dr. Harper. Now, mind you, it had been over a month since we found out that Sue had ovarian cancer, and I was thinking this was not good. When one has cancer one must move as quickly as possible to start treatment to have a better chance at beating the disease and hopefully finding oneself in remission. Nevertheless, the health care system is what it is—overworked to a degree—and the only way you will get immediate treatment is if you have a heart attack and are brought to the hospital in an ambulance. Well, we met Dr. Harper; he seemed like a very nice gentleman, and by my standards he was very honest and well-educated in his field.

Chapter 3
More Tests and the Fear Begins

Sue and I both believed that Dr. Harper would have read the Pap smear results and would elaborate on the type of cancer Sue had and would tell us what type of

chemotherapy Sue would receive, for how long, and what her chances were; no such luck. Dr. Harper said, "Since I am Sue's physician now and have the responsibility to treat her, we need to do another Pap smear, a vaginal exam, several blood tests, a CT scan, and a biopsy."

After hearing his list of tests and procedures I said to him, thinking, well, let's get them done today, "I am not trying to be rude or suggest that you do not know what you are doing, but should we not move as fast as possible to begin treatment?"

Dr. Harper said, "It makes sense to repeat the tests to make sure that the data is correct and we can plan a better plan of action."

Dr. Harper took my rather snotty comments in stride. "Tom," he said, "we need to determine what type of ovarian *cancer* Sue has. We also need to determine how far along the cancer has progressed, and based on the physical exam, it is possible that the cancer has already progressed into the abdominal cavity."

Sue and I were dumbfounded. I said, "But Dr. Harper, it has only been a little more than a month since we found the cancer."

He replied, "That is correct, but the original physician was a gynecologist, not a cancer expert. I know that you are both very concerned, as I am, but to make sure that we provide Sue with the best chance of remission, we need to perform all of the tests I talked about. The best I can do is push the staff to set up Sue's appointments as soon as possible."

I said, "Dr. Harper, I am glad that I picked an expert for my wife, and I understand where you are coming from. It appears that we have only one chance to save my wife."

His comment was, "That may be right, but let's wait and see."

After our conversation I was livid. This was the love of my life, and I would be dammed if I was going to let her die. Sue was quiet as we went to Dr. Harper's administrator and set up the appointments. We would have to wait another month before Sue could be treated. Sue and I walked out of the hospital hand in hand and went home. Sue went to bed early that night. I asked her if she was all right, and she said, "We can beat this," and started crying. I hugged her until she went to sleep.

I called her friend at work and told her what was going on with Sue and that she would need to take off several days in the next month. Sue's friends wished Sue well and said they would pray for Sue. The next morning was a Saturday, and I spent the entire day researching ovarian cancer as well as the different types of treatment, how it is staged, the potential for surgery, side effects of the treatment, the number of women who go into remission, the number of patients who do not respond to chemo, what the alternatives are, and the number of women who die within six months, a year, or live for three years or more, which is rare. I have to admit the research was agonizing for me.

It was a very busy day for me, but I had spent most of my life in medical research, and I was determined to learn as much about ovarian cancer as Dr. Harper.

After learning all of this information, I was devastated. This was a nasty form of cancer my wife had. Ovarian cancer is given a number based on all of the medical results from the tests that were taken. Sue was at the stage-four level, meaning that the cancer was very active and beginning to metastasize, which means it was spreading. It was the worst case in general.

In addition, we were also talking about possible progression to other organs of the body, and even with chemo, 60 percent of the women with this form of cancer will not reach remission and have the potential of dying from this type of cancer. Typically 60 percent of most of the patients will die in a year. To give people reading this book some hope, please remember that the data I am talking about was from three years ago and today the statistics maybe different.

Chapter 4
The Medical Results and
What Is Next

Sue and I sat in Dr. Harper's office side by side holding hands, waiting for the results of all of the tests and where we would go from there. Dr. Harper walked into the office and sat down and started to tell us about the information he had received from all the tests and what his plan was going to be.

Our first shock was that Sue did have a rare form of ovarian cancer called primary peritoneal cancer, a form of ovarian cancer that there is no cure for. Sue and I just stared at him, and I did not know what to say and just listened to my wife's death knell. Dr. Harper said that Sue needed surgery because the cancer had already spread from the endometrium to the abdomen. Dr. Harper said that the CT scan indicated that the amount of cancer in the abdominal cavity was significant, and the only chance of helping Sue to be able to receive chemo was a de-bulking procedure. I asked Dr. Harper to explain what a de-bulking procedure was because I knew Sue did not know what type of surgery that was.

Dr. Harper said, "In this case de-bulking is when the surgeon opens the abdominal cavity and uses a laser-type probe to destroy all of the tumors he can find to reduce the cancer burden. We have the ability to destroy cancer cells that are as small as one centimeter. Any cancer smaller than that will be taken care of by the chemo, we hope. The term cancer burden refers to the number of cancer cells that the immune system in our body can keep from dividing and growing in layman's terms. If this surgery is successful then the patient has a chance to receive chemotherapy to reduce the cancer burden even further so that the immune system can manage the cancer and slow down its progression. If the chemo is effective then the patient could be declared to be in remission."

Sue was overwhelmed by all of this medical jargon, and so I told Dr. Harper to go ahead and schedule the surgery. Sue and I left the hospital and went home. Up until this point Sue had managed the possible consequences of the disease very well, but when we got home she began to fall apart. I tried to console her and reminded her that we said we would beat this disease. Her family was advised by me of Sue's disease and how we had to treat it as quickly as possible in an effort to have Sue receive chemo and to have a chance to be in remission. I spoke to Sue's daughters separately as well about their mother's condition. Then it started—the phone calls, the good luck cards, the get well soon cards. It is enough to make one crazy. And yet the patient has to realize that her friends and family love her and don't know what else to do.

I explained to Sue everything Dr. Harper said to us in the office again so that Sue would have a better understanding of what the next month and a half would bring. I tried to keep her calm and continued to remind her often that if the surgery was successful she would receive chemo and had a good chance of going into remission. I tried as hard as I could to keep Sue thinking positive while inside I was afraid to consider the future because I knew the chance of Sue going into remission was less than 20 percent because the cancer had progressed so far up her abdomen.

The time had come, and Sue had her last day at work and took a medical leave of absence. The following week I packed her bag for her, and off to the hospital we went. Sue was admitted to the surgical floor. She was taken to her room and was told that the next day she would receive some tests prior to surgery and that if the tests were normal that Dr. Harper would perform the surgery the following day. I spent as much time with her as I was allowed that day and went home to an empty house and cried and prayed to God.

The next day I went to the hospital early. The guard tried to stop me and said, "You are too early for visiting hours."

I looked at him straight in the eye and said, "I am a doctor. I am not on the staff, but Dr. Harper is a friend of mine and invited me to observe a unique form of surgery that I intend to see. I did not come all the way from Connecticut to miss it."

The guard said to me, "Do you have any ID?"

I pulled out my business card, which said Dr. Thomas Lucas, and put my thumb over my credentials so the guard just saw Dr. and not the PhD. I started walking to the elevator and said again, "I can't be late. I have to scrub up."

The guard said, "Sorry, Doc, go ahead."

I said, "Thank you. I know you are just doing your job."

By now everyone must know that I would lie, steal, fight, or do anything I have to do to be beside my wife before she went into surgery. I walked into her room. Sue was prepped, but she said no one had told her of the results of the tests yet. I could see her IV was hanging by her side. Sue told me that the nurse already had given her a mild sedative, so I gave her a big kiss and a hug. I also gave her some flowers, which I have said before she loves, and sat by her holding her hand. I asked her if she was able to get any sleep the previous night. She said no, but the nurse was kind enough to give her some valium, so she could sleep.

I asked Sue again if anyone came into the room and discussed the results of the tests. Why ask again? Because I could tell Sue was still groggy from the valium. Sue was sensitive to most drugs. Sue said, "I did not see anybody, and I have not had breakfast."

I decided to look at her medical chart. I told Sue I was going to ask the nurse for her chart. Sue said to me, "They won't give that chart to you."

I said, "Would you like to make a bet?"

She laughed a little and said, "I forgot you are my doctor."

I said, "That is right. I know the jargon and can interpret the test results." I walked out of the room and returned in about two minutes and sat down next to Sue and told her what the results were. She seemed a little calmer when I told her that all of the test results for her surgery were normal and that she was ready to go.

I then asked Sue if she had seen Dr. Harper. She said, "He is in surgery. I am next." I asked her if she had seen the anesthesiologist and she said, "No, not yet."

I got up, walked out of her room, found her nurse, and said, "When can we expect the anesthesiologist?"

The nurse asked another nurse who said to me, "Who are you?"

I said, "I am Suzanne Gallen-Lucas's husband, and I am a doctor."

The head nurse said to me, "Oh, I am sorry, Doctor, we have to check who we are speaking to because a patient's history is private."

I said, "I am sorry I did not tell you I was a doctor right away."

The nurse said, "Oh, now that I know I will leave a note to the next shift that you are a doctor and can have Suzanne's chart anytime you want it."

I said, "Thank you."

Just a reminder to the people following this story—I have the right to call myself a doctor because I have a PhD and earned that title by completing my thesis. If nobody asks me what type of doctor I am, I do not have to tell them. The nurse said that the anesthesiologist should see Sue at about ten o'clock and she was scheduled for surgery at noon.

I said, "Noon? It is only six AM. I thought she was first on the list for surgery." The nurse told me that Dr. Harper had an emergency case and had to take another patient first. He said he had to push Sue's surgery back a couple of hours.

I looked at the nurse and said, "Well, Sue has not been given any food, just an IV."

The nurse said, "That is right. That is standard procedure. No food eight hours before surgery."

I said, "Well, did you know that Sue has hypoglycemia?"

She looked at me, looked at the chart, and said, "The chart does not say that."

I said, "Who took her history?"

She said, "Nurse Mary Beth last night."

I said, "Did nurse Mary Beth ask Sue these questions before or after she received valium?"

The nurse said, "After. We wanted her to get a good night's sleep."

I said, "Well, that was a nice thought, but did anybody ask Sue if she was sensitive to valium?"

The nurse said, "I am sure we did. That is procedure."

I said, "Well, she was probably not thinking because she is afraid and upset by her situation, so you probably need to call the attending Doc and tell him she is hypoglycemic." I then said, "I am sorry Sue did not tell you she was hypoglycemic, but I am sure you understand my wife's position. We will need another IV with D5W, dextrose, and water to make sure she does not get hypoglycemic. Low blood sugar is the last thing we need and have her faint before the surgery."

She said, "You're right, I will check with the attending doc."

I went back to Sue's room and told her what the story was and that the nurse was going to hang another IV with D5W. Sue looked at me and said, "I forgot to tell them that I have hypoglycemia."

I said, "That is why I am by your side, baby."

Sue looked at me with tears in her eyes and said, "What would I do without you?"

I said, "Don't worry, I will always be by your side, beautiful," and I gave her a hug and a kiss.

Time passed very slowly. I am not the type of person who just sits around and can be comfortable when my wife is going to have major surgery, so from time to time I would go outside for a cigarette or just walk the hallway. It was now noon, and the anesthesiologist came in and told us how he was going to treat Sue. I asked him if he was going to give her Versed, he looked at me and said, "How you know about Versed?"

I said, "I am a doctor and also have had surgery myself and it worked well for me."

Then it came, the proverbial question. I knew sooner or later it would. "What kind of a doctor are you?" he asked.

I said, "I am in medical research for a pharmaceutical company, and I am a Senior Director."

He said, "Any new drugs coming out soon?"

I said, "We will be releasing our data to the FDA in about a month, but the drug is confidential until we submit the data to the FDA."

He said, "I understand. Good luck with the research, and Sue, I will see you in the surgical suite," and he left the room. I did not lie; I just did not really answer his question. Oh well.

At twelve thirty they came to take Sue to the OR. I walked by her side until they would not let me go any farther. I gave her a kiss and told her I loved her and that I knew that everything would be fine. I got some lunch and went to the waiting room. Two hours passed and there was no sign of Dr. Harper yet. Two more hours passed by and I was now getting nervous. I walked to the nursing station and said, "Any word on Suzanne Gallen-Lucas's surgery yet?" They told me that she was still in surgery.

I said, "How long does de-bulking surgery take?"

The nurse said, "It depends on what they find and how much cancer is in her abdomen."

I was not a happy camper. My thought was the longer it took the more cancer they may have found. I was beside myself. I walked downstairs and into the hospital chapel. Now I have been in hospitals since I was thirteen years old but never walked into a hospital chapel before. It was empty, so I took a seat and started to pray to God.

"Dear God, please take Suzie by your hand and guide her surgeon through this surgery and help him to find every bit of cancer he can." I left the chapel and looked at my watch. It was now going on six hours. I went to the nursing station again and asked the nurse, "Has Dr. Harper finished my wife's surgery?"

The nurse said, "Oh yes, he left a message for you. He said to meet him at his office. He was changing his clothes and will be there in ten minutes."

"Thank God," I said to myself. "She made it through the surgery."

I walked over to his office and waited for him. He greeted me and said, "Let's sit down." We walked into his office. He sat behind his desk, and I sat on a chair directly in front of him.

Dr. Harper started talking by telling me the surgery went well. Sue was in recovery and would probably be in her room around eight o'clock. I just listened. He said that Sue had a significant amount to tumors all along her intestines. He said he was able to destroy as many as he could see.

I said, "What do you mean by that?"

He said, "With the technique we used today, which is significantly better than several years ago, we still cannot see any tumors smaller than a centimeter."

I just listened. "So that is the good news," he said.

"What is the bad news?" I said.

Dr. Harper said, "The cancer I could not see is still inside her. We will have to wait about a month for her to heal and then do a CT scan to see how active the remaining cancer is. If all is okay, we can start her on chemo." I started to tear up but held it back. Dr. Harper continued and said, "I am not that hopeful that we will find her to be status quo from the surgery. This form of cancer is rare and unpredictable. In a month she could be right back to where she was before the surgery.

"In addition, we took a blood sample before and after the surgery to measure her CA125 level. Do you know what that is?"

I said, "Yes, it is an antigen test to determine how much cancer is present. The higher the number the more cancer."

He said, "That is correct. Her value was four hundred. Usually when a woman's immune system can manage the cancer burden we will get a value of forty or less, but four hundred is not too bad. We've seen patients with values of one thousand and above."

There seemed to be some hope, I thought to myself. Dr. Harper finished up by saying, "It is a waiting game. The bottom line is she will probably not live beyond a year, which is my opinion based on my experience.

"I am sorry to say PPC is rare and we have not had much success in managing that form of cancer," he said.

I said to him, "How many cases have you treated?"

He said, "About eleven, which in the last five years is a lot."

Then I said, "How many of those patients are alive today?"

His comment was the longest survivor was three years.

I said, "Thank you for your report," and walked out the door, got into my car, and started to cry and cry, and I cried until I was exhausted. I regained my composure and drove home.

The next morning I called my secretary and told her I was taking the rest of the week off.

Sue's surgery was on a Tuesday, so that gave me Wednesday through Sunday to hope she might be released and be able to come home on Sunday. I called everybody in the family and let them know Sue came through the surgery without any additional problems and that if they wanted to see her they could come on Thursday to the hospital to say hello. I did not think it was the right time to tell Sue or her family that her chances of beating this form of cancer were very small.

The next morning I walked into Sue's room and saw her watching TV. There were tubes all over her body, nose, arm, and belly, but she said she had very little pain. I brought her a get well card, some flowers, and a set of rosary beads. I kissed her as best I could with all the tubes in the way and sat next to her and just tried to smile.

She was drowsy but finally looked at me and said, "Hi, baby." I asked her how she felt and she said, "It hurts a little, but they said by tomorrow I could probably drink some liquids." I asked her if she had seen Dr. Harper. She said no.

I said, "I saw him, and he said that the surgery went well and he was able to get rid of a significant amount of cancer." I told her as soon as she felt better we would discuss chemo with another doctor. Sue asked why another doctor. I said, "Because he is the head of the oncology division and he decides which chemo regimen would have the best chance of putting you into remission."

Dr. Harper is the surgeon and does not manage the chemo. When a patient has as much surgery as Sue had it is difficult to judge when the surgery will heal enough to be able to go home. I personally hate hospitals. In my career I have been in and out of so many hospitals I would rather stay home than go to another hospital, but that women in the bed in that hospital was my wife. You can be sure I was there every day holding her hand, talking with her, trying to keep her from thinking about the near future. Rather than a week it took Sue two weeks before she was able to come home. Her CA 125 was actually lower this time, which was positive, and she was eating well.

Chapter 5
The Plan

When Sue left the hospital they gave her an appointment for two weeks from then when we would see Dr. Burger, the chemo expert, and discuss where we go from there. While Sue was at home she just tried to relax and kept asking me about the chemo. I kept changing the subject but finally told her that she would receive a combination of two drugs that had the best chance of reducing the cancer level and that she could go into remission if it worked.

Two weeks passed very fast and we were at the hospital waiting to see Dr. Burger. His nurse took Sue's vital signs and left us sitting in an examination room. This older gentlemen enter the room and said, "Hello, I am Dr. Burger. Your vital signs are good, and the results of the surgery indicated that you still have some cancer.

"I am planning to put your wife on a regimen of platinum and cis-platinum. It is your best chance of maybe going into remission. We start next week."

He was ready to get up and walk out when I stopped him and said, "Excuse me, Dr. Burger, I am Dr. Lucas, Suzanne's husband, and I have some questions if you don't mind."

He looked at me and said, "My nurse can explain that."

I said, "I would like you to explain the procedure."

He said, "It will be a five-month course of chemo. You will come to the hospital once a week to receive the chemo. You will spend most of the day at the hospital during that period.

"When you go home, just try and relax. If you get any side effects from the chemo, call us and we will prescribe meds for you."

He was ready to walk out of the room again and I said, "Why will Sue only receive the chemo once a month?"

Dr. Burger said, "The drug Sue is receiving takes up to a month to have its effect. As time goes on Sue will feel the effects of the chemo sooner each month."

"What kind of side effects can we expect?" I said.

Dr. Burger said, "We will give you a list of side effects you can expect."

I said, "Such as?" I was not giving up until I get all the info I could.

Something for everybody who is reading this book—ask every question you can think of. Some doctors have the attitude that they are talking to a layman who would not understand what he is saying anyway. If you do not understand the doctor's comment, tell him to phrase it so that you can understand what he means. Let's face it, he is getting paid! Dr. Burger said, "Some nausea, vomiting, some pain. It is spelled out in the material we give you." I asked Dr. Burger what Sue's chance of going into remission was. He blankly said, "Less than 25 percent."

Dr. Burger said, "As we continue with the chemo you will visit my resident doctor every two weeks and can tell him how you are managing." He said goodbye and good luck and walked out the door.

I turned to Sue and said, "He has the worst bedside manner I have ever encountered. Let's get the paperwork from the nurse and go home."

During Sue's fight for life she had five courses of chemotherapy over a period of six months in total, starting from the end of 2005 to the middle of 2007. The most effective treatment they had to offer was platinum and cis-platinum. That would be her chemotherapy and her best chance to go into remission. The nurse took Sue's vital signs, gave Sue some juice, and gave her some medicine to make sure Sue was not allergic to the chemo.

The chemo center was very nice. Each patient had a TV to watch. The nurses were friendly and checked up on Sue every hour. They asked her if she needed anything, and I got to sit right next to my wife. The procedure took almost five hours. They have to give the patient the medication slowly. We are really talking about giving somebody poison. This process would occur every month once a week until Sue received the full course of chemo.

As the months went by, Sue started getting some side effects—vomiting, nausea, and pain. I would call up the hospital and ask for the resident doc, and he would prescribe meds for Sue. The meds helped, but Sue still was not herself. During that time Sue's surgery healed, and she was able to walk around our house a little, watch TV, eat some good food, not much though, and tried to relax.

As time went on Sue started getting stomach pains. Sue could not go to the bathroom, would vomit, or would be nauseated, all typical side effects from the chemo. I called the resident physician as soon as Sue started getting repeat side effects.

The resident doctor wrote scripts for several more drugs for the side effects. The resident was very understanding and kind. As time went on to the second and third month the side effects came more quickly and Sue was very uncomfortable to say the least. I had to take a leave of absence from work because someone needed to be by Sue's side almost 24/7.

By the first of November Sue was receiving more and more morphine on a daily basis and still little relief from the pain from the chemo. Sue quite often had this very painful feeling emanating from her distended abdomen, which radiated to her lower back. I would give her another dose of morphine, followed by Ativan for the anxiety and a compazine suppository for the nausea and potential vomiting.

As an aside, there are approximately eight generic names for morphine, with various times to peak. In layman's terms, that is when the drug has its strongest effect. Then there is the duration of action—that is how long the effect will last—and of course the typical morphine side effects. Morphine works well but not without significant side effects. As the chemo wears off, the patient begins to feel a little better just before the next course of chemo. Depending on the type of chemo the patient receives, he or she can have more or fewer side effects. It also depends on the patient.

Sue, for instance, had a fair tolerance for pain, which in the beginning of the chemo made life a little easier for her to manage. It was a tough six months, but the course of chemo was finally over and we had an appointment with the doctor. In the oncologist's office we were both worried about what he would say. Dr. Burger said the chemotherapy was finished and now it was a waiting game, which implied the chemo was going to work. All Sue's blood tests indicated that the cancer burden was down and there was no sign of metastasis.

The physician's comment to us was, "If Sue has no more symptoms for the next six months then we can declare her in remission." We walked out of the office a little more relaxed and went home. As the effects of the chemo were beginning to wear off, Sue was able to sleep better. She began moving around the house again, did some small chores, read books, and took a walk from time to time. Her friends would come and visit her. The children stopped by, and she would talk to her friends at work. Life almost seemed normal. Sue was not in much pain. She ate small meals because of the surgery, which had left massive scars in her abdomen. Sue would smile at me from time to time, which was wonderful, but I knew that inside she was anxious to find out if she was in remission. We got a break from all the stress and anxiety for fifty-eight days. Then the roof caved in. Sue's stomach was getting a little bigger, so I called the doctor. The doctor said that the swelling could be expected because of the surgery and leftover fluids.

Chapter 6
The Results and Where We Go from Here

Sue's test results indicated that the cancer was stable at a CA125 value of forty.

It was time to visit the doctor again. We sat and waited in his office for about a half an hour. Both of us were nervous as to what the physician was going to say. When Dr. Burger walked in he did not say hello. He just spouted out that the chemotherapy did not work.

I said to him, "Based on what data?" He said, "Well, her CA125 level should be lower, and it has gone up a couple of points."

I said to him, "Dr. Burger, it is common for that value to fluctuate from time to time. Next week it could be a value of twenty. How can you be so sure the chemo had no effect at all?"

He just looked at me and said, "Oh, I forgot you are some kind of a doctor."

I got very mad and said, "That is right I have a MS degree, a PhD, and a MD in cardiovascular medicine and have several years of research experience. I also took a sixty-hour course in oncology at Harvard Medical School."

The MD was a lie, but the other degrees and the oncology course were true. Then Dr. Burger said, "And in addition to the CA125, Sue is two days short of six months."

My comment was, "Okay, so the chemo did not work one hundred percent, but based on my knowledge she is a good candidate for another course of chemo."

Sue turned green; she did not want to go through that torture again.

The doctor repeated himself and said, "She is two days short of being in remission."

I said, "Two days seems to me to be an arbitrary number."

He just looked at me and said, "We gave her the best care and chance we could and the most up-to-date treatment available. There is nothing else we can give her. Here is a script for some pain meds. Just take her home and let her die in peace."

I got up from my chair and closed his office door and I said to him in a very angry voice, "So you are just going to let her die after just one course of chemo because she was two days short of your six-month goal and having some signs of the cancer being active again? There must be some new drugs that the hospital is researching. Maybe Sue would be a good candidate for a different kind of chemo."

His immediate comment was no. I said, "How do you know? Have you researched any new studies being conducted outside of your domain?"

He just looked at me and said, "Do you know how many years of experience with cancer patients I have?"

I said, "I do not know, and I do not care. You are here to help patients give it their best, and come up with other possible treatments that may be available."

He looked at me and said, "I am sorry," and walked out of his office.

Sue was now crying and scared. I was so angry because I never give up, especially when it comes to my wife or family. I hugged Sue and said, "Let's go home. I will find out who would be a good oncologist nearby and we will get a second opinion." We went home, and Sue took a nap. In a half hour I got the name of an oncologist who came highly recommended and set up an appointment.

For the next week Sue was very quiet and alone because I had to travel for work. I knew she was very depressed and scared, so I tried to call her twice a day. I do not know if it helped or not.

Chapter 7
We Get a Second Opinion

The week ended, and on Monday we had another appointment with a Dr. Rogers, who was retired but was an oncologist and well respected. He had Sue's chart and we spoke with him. Unlike the other jackass, he was more sympathetic, but his comment was the same. There was nothing that medicine could do for my wife.

Sue decided to put her last will and testament together and her living will as well. I did the best to not allow Sue to see me crying. When I felt it coming over me I went into the bathroom and turned on the fan so Sue would not hear me crying, but when I came out of the bathroom Sue just looked at my face and said, "You were crying." All I could do was walk over to her and hug her and tell her how much I loved her. The next couple of weeks were very bad. Sue started to feel fluid building up in her stomach. I told her she had ascities. It is common when cancer metastasizes from one area of the body to another. In this case the cancer was spreading from the upper vaginal area to the intestines and slowly killing or blocking the intestines, hence the fluid buildup (ascities). From time to time I had to take Sue to a local hospital and they would with draw the fluid from her stomach, sometimes as much as two quarts. When the fluid was gone she felt better. I kept in touch with the surgeon who did the surgery on Sue before she received the chemo. He had left the first hospital Sue received her chemo at and was at another hospital as a director of gynecologic surgery as well as vaginal cancer. He was very well educated, well liked, caring, and would not give up on his patients unless they were too far gone.

Sue had to go to our local hospital every three weeks to get the fluid removed. The nurses and techs were wonderful. There was a period of time when Sue was so sick that she had to be hospitalized again at the local hospital close to where we lived. A GI doc who approved the removal of fluid from Sue's abdomen said to me, after reading her history, "You do realize that your wife is dying and removing this fluid every three weeks is a waste of time and your money."

I said to him, "So you feel we should just take her home and let her die."

He looked at me and said yes.

I said, "Release my wife now. We are leaving this hospital, and you will never see her again because you don't care." He tried to argue with me that I was expecting a miracle and I said, "Yes, and if none of you experts can come up with another form of chemo for my wife to try then I will." He just looked at me like I was some kind of fruitcake.

When we got home I had to tell the family that the chemo did not work and the doctors gave Sue maybe two more months before she would die. I was working part time, so Sue had a nurse come by every day for vital signs. Sue's middle daughter came to live with us so that Sue could have company and to give her pain meds when she needed them. The family stopped by to see Sue and talk to her and told her they would pray for her. I told them not to discuss Sue's death at all.

Sue got worse day by day. She could not eat and was losing weight. She could not walk to the bathroom by herself anymore. She slept about fifteen hours a day. Due to Sue's condition, I told her to sleep on the big couch downstairs, which she found more comfortable compared to our bed upstairs. I did not want to take a chance that if we slept together that I might bump into her when I turned in bed.

I also went out and bought a children's call system so if I was asleep and Sue needed something I would hear her and wake up and go downstairs and take care of her needs. Sue was still filling up with fluids, and her friends and family were just waiting for her to die. On the other hand, I, her husband, was not going to give her up. The family thought that I was nuts and that Sue should be in hospice care. They tried to console me and said to me, "Well, you had nine great years with Sue. It could have been less." I said, "Sue and I have a twenty-year contract for marriage," and walked away.

The next day I left my job for good and explained to my boss the situation. He understood and said, "Good luck, Tom." By now Sue needed to be in a hospital. She had lost a lot of weight, could not eat, and just slept a lot. The nurse and social worker would come and visit Sue twice a week. They all agreed that was the appropriate way to go, so that Sue could die in peace. I said, "No, if my wife is going to die it will be at home." So the nursing team set up a hospital bed in our den. Sue was more comfortable laying on the hospital bed rather than one of our beds or the couch, which could not be raised or lowered.

We discussed giving Sue her pain meds and who I should call when Sue passed away, and when the nurse felt that I could take care of Sue they were ready to leave. Before they left I noticed something that was missing—an IV for water because Sue had a hard time swallowing. I asked the nurse where the IV was, and she said to me that it was not necessary since Sue would probably die in a day or so due to her condition.

I said to the nurse, "We do not know that for sure."

The nurse just looked at me and said, "I know this is very hard on you," but I immediately said, "No, but it is illegal to leave a dying patient without water. It is against the law."

She checked with her associate and they agreed that I was right. You see, hospice is set up to have the patient die as soon as possible without feeling pain. The nurse set up an IV, and they left. Now Sue's daughter and I just had to see if we could get Sue to eat liquids and give her the pain meds.

Well, as I said, I never give up, so while Sue was comfortable I spent the next couple of days reading every new form of chemo being used for PPOC I could find. I looked through dozens of medical journals with new thoughts on arresting cancer. I said to myself, "Would radiation work? How about radiation and chemo?" but there was little, if any, information on the type of cancer Sue had.

I started calling every research center in the United States that was conducting studies on different types of cancer to find out if their drugs would work on Sue. I knew we could not save Sue from dying, but I had hope we could extend her life a little longer.

Eventually I gave up my search on new drugs, combination drugs, different kinds of research studies, voodoo, praying to God every day—nothing was going to make a difference with the type of cancer Sue had. Then a thought hit me, "How do our bodies take care of themselves when they are invaded by, say, bacteria or a virus? How does the immune system work? I started reading again about how our white cells work when we have an infection. What do T cells do, how do T cells kill a virus? After several days of reading, I came across an article that said, "Live healthier, eat right, and limit getting sick by busting your level of anti-oxidants."

That was right. I remembered reading about anti-oxidants in college and graduate school. I went to the library and got every copy of any medical journal or chemical journal that had an article on the function of anti-oxidants. Where do we get anti-oxidants from, you might ask. From fruits and vegetables, I said to myself, and green tea. I hit the jackpot. I researched the fruits and vegetables highest in anti-oxidants. I decided to develop a recipe of food with high levels of anti-oxidants. Sue was status quo and was able to eat some Jell-O-type food. So I decided to go to a place like GNC and get pills with green tea. Then I picked up the proper green vegetables like spinach, broccoli, and any colored or green fruit that would have antioxidants in it.

I cut up all the fruits and vegetables and put them in a blender, added the green tea, and mixed it up into a smooth liquid. Then I tasted it was bitter, so I added some sugar, just a bit, so that it did not taste so bad. Then I gave it to Sue to drink.

Sue did not like the taste and had a problem swallowing it down, so I made the concoction smoother by adding more water, and I made Sue drink it three times a day for a week. When Sue could manage the drink, I increased the dose by double. A week later I pushed the dose as high as I could and Sue was still able to manage it. Meanwhile Sue started to feel a little better. Sue was beginning to talk again, and she did not sleep as much. Sue was going to the bathroom again in a potty, believe it or not. I did not care if the drink was making a difference or not. All I cared about was that Sue was feeling better.

It had now been a month since the nurse said to me Sue would probably die in a couple of days. One day Sue said to me, "Tom, I think I can sleep on the couch again. I do not feel bad at all."

I took Sue's vital signs, and they were all normal. I told the nurse to get rid of the hospital bed and that she did not need to come back. I could take care of my own wife. I was crying at the thought that Sue might live a little longer.

We had a wonderful Christmas, believe it or not, because Sue was still alive. She was comfortable for almost six weeks.

Chapter 8
Sue Begins to Slide Downhill Again

After Christmas I called Dr. Harper. He did not believe that Sue was still alive and set up an appointment for Sue. We went to the hospital, and Dr. Harper examined Sue. Her abdomen had only a little bit of fluid, her vital signs were good, and the CA 125 was twenty-eight, meaning the cancer burden was less. Dr. Harper could not believe what he was seeing. I told him what I did, and he was amazed. He said to me, "Let's wait another month and see how she feels then." We came back in a month and everything was stable. Dr. Harper told us he was experimenting with patients who have PPOC with a drug called Taxol and wanted to give it to Sue. We both looked at each other and said, "Great, let's do it."

Sue was scheduled for chemo again once a week for four months. This chemo had fewer side effects, and Sue was relatively comfortable at home but still needed some pain meds to manage. I thought about going back to work but decided to stay at home with Sue. The chemotherapy was initiated. We lived rather far from the hospital where Dr. Harper worked at. I decided to sell our house because the ride to the hospital was an hour away. I wanted the trip to the hospital to be as easy as possible for Sue. We moved to a new neighborhood after selling our house, and the ride was only about twenty minutes.

We lived in a two-bedroom apartment that was very nice and convenient with a pharmacy nearby for Sue's scripts. We were also closer to my sons and Sue's family so Sue could get to see her family and friends more often.

Well, until Sue's third month everything was going fine, and then Sue started to get ascites again. Since we were near Dr. Harper's hospital we decided to get the extraction of Sue's fluid at Dr. Harper's hospital. The nurses were friendly, and the tech was great at removing the abdominal fluid without causing Sue a lot of pain, and Dr. Harper would always come down from his office to see Sue. During our routine visit after Sue had three months of chemo Dr. Harper took me aside and said, "Tom, the chemo is not working." He showed me an X-ray of her stomach, which was filled with fluid, and her CA125 was back to forty again. Sue was feeling week and beginning to vomit and had nausea again.

I asked Dr. Harper if it was worth finishing the last course of chemo, and he said, "No, Tom, it will not help and only give Sue more pain." By now I trusted him and I agreed. I asked Dr. Harper how much time Sue would have left, and he said, "Who can tell with the way she previously responded to your herbal treatment?"

Dr. Harper told me to take her home and watch her and keep him up to date. We went home.

Chapter 9
I Take Sue Home to Die

Living in an apartment made it easier for me to take care of Sue. Sue would stay on the couch most of the day, and at night she slept in our bed. I slept in the next room, and any time Sue called me for anything I was right there. Sue was getting weak and still losing weight. In the morning I would dress her and wash her hands and face. I would help her move to the couch and turn the TV on for her. She had the remote, but honestly, she would fall asleep in about a half hour because she was so weak. The nurse came to see her every other day and check her vital signs

As time went on Sue told me that whenever she ate her stomach just got bloated, no matter if it was soup or just some Jell-O, so in essence she really was not getting any food. I called Dr. Harper and told him what was going on with her. He said, "I think it is time to put a tube in Sue's stomach with a bag attached." I asked him to explain to me his concern.

Dr. Harper said that Sue's intestines were in spasm due to the cancer taking over any space available within her abdomen. He said, "I will prescribe a muscle relaxant and see if it helps to get the food from her stomach to drain into the intestines." We gave Sue her new drug three times a day, and after a week we realized that it was not having an effect.

So off to the hospital we went again, and the surgery was finished in an hour. Sue stayed in the hospital for just a day and then they released her. When we got back home, I could take off her bandages. Sue had a tube in the side of her stomach that led to a plastic bag. For a few days I had to change her small bandage and put another one in its place until the hole around the stomach tube closed up. From time to time I would have to clean out Sue's bag and the tube in her stomach. I forgot to tell you that the tube in her stomach also had a bypass tube. One tube was always in her stomach, and the other tube came out of her stomach. That tube was about six inches long and closed at the end. From time to time I had to open that tube and extract liquid from her stomach that was backing up from her intestines. The system worked well, and Sue could get some food into her intestines from time to time.

The next problem we encountered was that the food took a long time to move through the small and large intestines to reach ultimately the rectum. This meant that Sue could not move her bowels without a suppository. So from day to day it was feed Sue, clean her tube out, reduce the fluid in her stomach, which caused pain, wait a day or so, and give Sue a suppository. This lifestyle for Sue lasted a month until Sue told me she was in a lot of pain. I then had to give Sue a shot of morphine twice a day. This helped Sue manage the pain for a week or two and then the pain got worse, so then it was a shot of morphine three times a day. Sue was losing weight at a rate of three pounds a week. The last time I weighed Sue she was eighty-nine pounds. My beautiful wife looked like a stick. Her arms were like a skeletons arms, and her face was sunken in. Sue slept more each day. I called the nurse who came over to our house and told her she did not have to come to see Sue anymore to take her vital signs, that I could handle that.

I knew Sue's time was almost up, so I called her family, and day by day her family and friends came by to see their mother or friend for the last time. Most of the time Sue was out of it because the morphine dose was as high as the doctor would let me give to Sue without being in the hospital. Most of the time now Sue was asleep, and from time to time I had to check to see if the love of my life was still breathing. When it was time for me to go to sleep I usually cried myself to sleep knowing that my wife would not be with me much longer. That day finally came. Sue was asleep on the couch. I was watching some TV, when all of a sudden Sue managed to sit up on her own.

I said to Sue, "Are you okay? Do you need more morphine?"

Sue said to me, "Tommy, I cannot take the pain anymore. I want to give up and die."

I went over to Sue and hugged her. I must have kissed her at least ten times, and I was crying, but Sue was so out of it that she did not even realize that I was crying like a baby. I called for an ambulance and called Dr. Harper and he called the hospice ward and told them one of his patients was coming in.

Chapter 10
Hospice

I got to the hospital at the same time the ambulance did. They took Sue up to the hospice ward, and I was right by her side. They put Sue in the hospital bed, changed her clothes, and hung two IV bags, one for D5W and one for morphine.

They also had a monitor for her vital signs, pulse, heart rate, and blood pressure. Sue looked comfortable. I sat next to her and handed her the rosary. I called her daughters and told them where their mother was and they came by and sat with me next to their mother. I told them it was useless to try and talk to her because Sue was now receiving six hundred milligrams of morphine.

The goal of the hospice ward was to make the patient as comfortable as possible so that the patient could pass away in peace. I spent every day with Sue by her side, from ten o'clock in the morning until six at night, and then I would go home to an empty apartment and just cry. The next day I would go back to the hospital and I would hug her and kiss her, and I even brought her some flowers. Sue did not even know I was there. I made arrangements for Sue's last rites and with the funeral home. After a week in the hospice room, I noticed that Sue was not moving, her eyes were almost closed, and she was having a hard time breathing. Her chest would heave from time to time; it was very difficult for me to watch the love of my life die slowly. I cherished every minute I was by her side.

The next morning when I went to see Sue, I walked into the room and it seemed like Sue may have died the previous night, but I could not believe that could happen without the hospital calling me. I walked over to Sue and touched her head. It was cold. Her legs were cold, and her lips were blue. I gave her a kiss and got no response. A couple of seconds later it occurred,

Sue took a deep breath, to my surprise, but then I remembered that when a patient is very close to death they have what is called death rails. Basically the body is trying to breathe but most of the systems in the body are closing down, so it is hard to breathe.

I sat next to Sue and held her hand, and from time to time her chest would heave. I put my mouth next to Sue's ear and said, "Sue, it is okay, you can let go now; I will take care of our children." I do not know if Sue heard me or not. That night I got a call from the hospital that Sue had passed away at one o'clock in the morning. The next morning I entered her room and walked over to Sue's bed.

I looked at my baby for a minute or two. Then I caressed her hair a couple of times. I leaned down and gave my wife my last kiss and said goodbye to her. I told her I would love her forever and would never forget our life together and that I would never find another woman like her because she was one of a kind. To this day on her birthday I put flowers next to her urn, and I write her a birthday card.

The end.

Letters and Some Poems to My Wife, Suzanne

How Was I to Know

How was I to know when we first met that she
was the one, my soul mate to be kept?
How was I to know that when I was near her that
my heart would skip a beat and flutter rapidly?
How was I to know when we were walking hand
in hand and the sun shone down on her beautiful
hair that I would see an angel in disguise?
How was I to know that her beautiful face and
magic eyes would compromise even Helen of
Troy's well-known legion?

It came to be that she married me, and I learned much more than I could see.

The softness of her skin was gentle to the touch; her form was molded as such that no matter how she dressed she looked like a celebrity to me. No makeup was needed from morning till night, she shone like a star on a clear, dark night

Her nature was calm and expressed class, her intellect was refined, and oh that smile, it was all mine, to me, for me, as no other had before me

Her passion was a fire in a rage, out of control, and never spent when it came to loving me

Her caring and honesty was directed to me without a doubt, our relationship was cemented, and together we would be for all eternity.

And so I lived on happily with my dream woman beside me, through the ups and downs of life we managed it all.

I had gained a best friend, a loving wife, and on my knees I thanked God for sending me a soul mate

The Rose of My L9fe

Raised as a gentleman, for those were the times, I married too young and found out from behind, life is never perfect. I surely was not. I tried very hard, but the old door was locked. I never really had the proverbial key.

Divorce is so bad, filled with pain and hate; I reached for the bottle and then met my fate. Savaging here and there, trying to squelch my despair. The children I knew I had to live for, and so I found the strength to move on once more, and the bottle, it was gone.

Now angels come from time to time, I was told, and say a few words and then they move on. But this one left a surprise for me. She said, "It is the rose of your life, care for it, nurture it, feed it with love,

Only you can save it, it has been abandoned before. Give it life and you will be surprised at how rich you will feel and how alive."

I held it gently and placed it in the sun; I watered it and then some. To my surprise, it did not die. How long can a flower last once taken from the vine? Now love and caring is what it wanted, and thorns around its stalk were needed no more.

It was my friend from day till night. It gave me a smile and much delight. It was mine to care for with love indeed. Not a day went by that I did not see the rose of my life. And then one day it was very pale, and withered and died. I cried. And the angel heard my tears and returned and said, "Her time was up. You did very well. Now take you turn and live life well." I knew not what she meant.

I thought to myself, this must be a dream, I must wake up. But I was awake, and so I laughed at my fantasy and went to work as always. And on that day, to my surprise, I met a woman with beautiful eyes. Her smile was so bright you could see it at night; a face so divine like it was just picked from a vine. Her stalk was perfect, not one little thorn. We became best friends and coveted each other's needs from heart to heart.

And then we agreed our life should be as one, to have and hold, to love and share, to support when in despair. Happy and content, we lived our life as was meant. Thirteen years of bliss is what we had, and then one day she fell away with me by her side, and I cried. And the angel returned and said, "Do not weep, she is here." "But where?" I said. "I see her not," and she gave me a flower, and in my hand was the love of my life, and I caressed it so and kissed it, and the angel said, "You have lost her not. She will be with you until you time runs out, and then you will both be free to live all eternity as spirit and soul together," and I cried.

Dedicated to the rose of my life, my wife, Suzanne, forever.

Thank You for Being My Wife

With tears in my eyes and sorrow within my heart I write this thank you note to the woman of my life. Until I met you, a woman with class to me was just a woman with money, smothered with jewels and furs who forgot how to drive a car and looked down on others.

You were my epitome of class. You approached strangers with a smile and said hello. When you walked down the street men would glance. They could see your confidence in the way you walked, and yet you still said hello.

You were proud of who you were and how hard you worked to get there, and yet you never looked down at others. Diamonds were nice, but you never needed them. Furs were lovely, but you never needed them. You shined because you had a heart of gold.

Just a high school graduate you would remain, but your self-educated intelligence everyone could see in your common sense, in your use of vocabulary at a spelling bee. Your manners were polished, your morals were clear, and you attracted attention as soon as you smiled and uttered just a few words, hello

Age affects us all, but you were divine. My partner, my friend, my support, my lover indeed,

I have to admit you were perfect for me. Thank you for being my wife.

Things Happen for a Reason

Dear God,

I send this letter to you with my deepest respect. I do not pretend to understand some of the things that happen around me, or in our world, or why people kill each other, and why there is not more caring and understanding in this world, or how the universe became, or what or where is heaven.

As a scientist I can reiterate the data and experiments that men have produced over the years to try and unlock the mysteries of the world, but we do not have all the answers, and so at some point at least I have to say there must be a higher power.

There is a common phrase that my wife used often, whether the happening was good or bad. I believe you know her and the phrase, "Things happen for a reason."

When I was thirteen, I was an altar boy at Saint Anthony's school in Queens, New York. I had been picked to serve at a funeral for a nineteen-year-old boy who died in the very beginning of the Vietnam War. I stood by the casket with three other altar boys with a blessed candle in my hand while the priest blessed the casket and prayed for eternal life in heaven. The wife of the solider was sitting in the front pew with a very young baby in her arms, and when the priest finished his prayers he walked over to her and said, "God has taken him for a reason. He is in a better place." The young women started crying and said, "But he will never meet his daughter, and how will I support myself without him?" and she continued to cry. She was so distraught that I started crying with her and looked up to heaven and said, "This does not make any sense. Why not take a bad guy?"

When one of my best friends from childhood died not long ago, I had the same thought. He was a loving husband and a great dad to his four sons. He never hurt anyone, and he was only fifty-nine years old. His wife now has the task of raising her young men by herself. She was devoted to him and now has to move because their finances did not allow her to stay in their home of over twenty years.

She works in a cancer hospital and helps people. Why so soon, God? I may understand the medical reason that he passed away, but why him?

Just why so soon? What is he doing now with you that could be better than to love and care for his family and lead a good life? Since I knew him for forty years, I believe that his lifestyle was akin to the lives we are all supposed to live according to the Bible.

Now I know some people may think that I am arrogant to question God. I am not being disrespectful, although my faith is not as strong as it was when I was younger. Seeing too much bloodshed by God's people does not make much sense to me.

My first name is Thomas. God, I am sure you know that, and I am also sure that you have heard me say sometimes I follow in Thomas the Apostle's footsteps when I say, "I am doubting Thomas." As a scientist there are so many questions without answers and not just questions about people on Mars, but more mundane questions like hatred, killing, and breaking every one of the Ten Commandments. I would have thought by now that there would have been some divine intervention to help set your flock on the right path and encourage love.

Again, I am not being disrespectful. You know me well. I just do not understand. I am sure it is beyond me, but when you made me with so much love to give and caring I thought, "Well, I cannot be so special" and that there must be more people like me. Together we may have been able to make a difference, and I think some people are, but changing is so slow that we need more people like that.

My wife was one of those people. She was a great mother and always supported her children. She raised them to be loving and caring. She followed the Bible as best as she could. Remember that none of us are perfect. You took her from me recently, as you know. She made me a better person. We were best friends and soul mates together. We had similar thoughts on how to raise our children. Now I have my two sons to advise, three step-daughters to advise, and three grandchildren to advise.

Why me, dear God? Why break my heart by taking her from me at a young age when I was at the happiest time of my life with her? I am not sure if I am strong enough to handle this task by myself. They say the good die young, and Sue said things happen for a reason. I am at a loss to understand your divine ways. If you could shed some light on this I would be most appreciative. I know there are billions of people in the world and I am only one of them, little me, but if you could, maybe send one of your messengers to shed some light on this issue for me. I would be glad to share it with so many others out there who I believe feel the same as me. If I have been arrogant to think that God has the time to stop for me then I do truly apologize.

Sincerely,

Thomas